I0706871

Today's Goal ______________   (M) (T) (W) (T) (F) (S) (S)

Muscle Group Focus ___________   Weight _________   Date/Time ___________

Stretch ◯   Warm-Up ______________________________________

Strength Training

Exercise		Set 1	Set 2	Set 3	Set 4	Set 5	Set 6
	Reps						
	Weight						
	Reps						
	Weight						
	Reps						
	Weight						
	Reps						
	Weight						
	Reps						
	Weight						
	Reps						
	Weight						
	Reps						
	Weight						
	Reps						
	Weight						
	Reps						
	Weight						

Cardio

Exercise	Calories	Distance	Time

Water Intake ________________

Cooldown ________________

Feeling ☆ ☆ ☆ ☆ ☆

Notes

Today's Goal ______________ Ⓜ Ⓣ Ⓦ Ⓣ Ⓕ ⬤ ⬤

Muscle Group Focus __________ Weight ________ Date/Time __________

Stretch ◯ Warm-Up _______________________________

Strength Training

Exercise		Set 1	Set 2	Set 3	Set 4	Set 5	Set 6
	Reps						
	Weight						
	Reps						
	Weight						
	Reps						
	Weight						
	Reps						
	Weight						
	Reps						
	Weight						
	Reps						
	Weight						
	Reps						
	Weight						
	Reps						
	Weight						
	Reps						
	Weight						
	Reps						
	Weight						

Cardio

Exercise	Calories	Distance	Time

Water Intake _______________

Cooldown _______________

Feeling ☆ ☆ ☆ ☆ ☆

Notes

Today's Goal _____________ Ⓜ Ⓣ Ⓦ Ⓣ Ⓕ ⬤S ⬤S

Muscle Group Focus __________   Weight ________   Date/Time __________

Stretch ◯   Warm-Up _______________________

Strength Training

Exercise		Set 1	Set 2	Set 3	Set 4	Set 5	Set 6
	Reps						
	Weight						
	Reps						
	Weight						
	Reps						
	Weight						
	Reps						
	Weight						
	Reps						
	Weight						
	Reps						
	Weight						
	Reps						
	Weight						
	Reps						
	Weight						

Cardio

Exercise	Calories	Distance	Time

Water Intake _______________

Cooldown _______________

Feeling ☆ ☆ ☆ ☆ ☆

Notes

Today's Goal _____________ Ⓜ Ⓣ Ⓦ Ⓣ Ⓕ ⬤S ⬤S

Muscle Group Focus ___________   Weight _________   Date/Time ___________

Stretch ◯   Warm-Up _________________________________

Strength Training

Exercise		Set 1	Set 2	Set 3	Set 4	Set 5	Set 6
	Reps						
	Weight						
	Reps						
	Weight						
	Reps						
	Weight						
	Reps						
	Weight						
	Reps						
	Weight						
	Reps						
	Weight						
	Reps						
	Weight						
	Reps						
	Weight						
	Reps						
	Weight						

Cardio

Exercise	Calories	Distance	Time

Water Intake _________________

Cooldown _______________

Feeling ☆ ☆ ☆ ☆ ☆

Notes

Today's Goal ________________   Ⓜ Ⓣ Ⓦ Ⓣ Ⓕ Ⓢ Ⓢ

Muscle Group Focus __________   Weight _________   Date/Time __________

Stretch ◯   Warm-Up ____

Strength Training

Exercise		Set 1	Set 2	Set 3	Set 4	Set 5	Set 6
	Reps						
	Weight						
	Reps						
	Weight						
	Reps						
	Weight						
	Reps						
	Weight						
	Reps						
	Weight						
	Reps						
	Weight						
	Reps						
	Weight						
	Reps						
	Weight						
	Reps						
	Weight						

Cardio

Exercise	Calories	Distance	Time

Water Intake ________________

Cooldown ________________

Feeling ☆ ☆ ☆ ☆ ☆

Notes

Today's Goal ___________ Ⓜ Ⓣ Ⓦ Ⓣ Ⓕ 🅢 🅢

Muscle Group Focus ___________ Weight _______ Date/Time _________

Stretch ◯ Warm-Up _______________________________

Strength Training

Exercise		Set 1	Set 2	Set 3	Set 4	Set 5	Set 6
	Reps						
	Weight						
	Reps						
	Weight						
	Reps						
	Weight						
	Reps						
	Weight						
	Reps						
	Weight						
	Reps						
	Weight						
	Reps						
	Weight						
	Reps						
	Weight						
	Reps						
	Weight						
	Reps						
	Weight						

Cardio

Exercise	Calories	Distance	Time

Water Intake _______________

Cooldown _______________

Feeling ☆ ☆ ☆ ☆ ☆

Notes

Today's Goal ______________ Ⓜ Ⓣ Ⓦ Ⓣ Ⓕ ⬤S ⬤S

Muscle Group Focus __________   Weight _______   Date/Time __________

Stretch ◯   Warm-Up ______________________________

Strength Training

Exercise		Set 1	Set 2	Set 3	Set 4	Set 5	Set 6
	Reps						
	Weight						
	Reps						
	Weight						
	Reps						
	Weight						
	Reps						
	Weight						
	Reps						
	Weight						
	Reps						
	Weight						
	Reps						
	Weight						
	Reps						
	Weight						
	Reps						
	Weight						
	Reps						
	Weight						

Cardio

Exercise	Calories	Distance	Time

Water Intake ______________

Cooldown ______________

Feeling ☆ ☆ ☆ ☆ ☆

Notes

Today's Goal ______________ Ⓜ Ⓣ Ⓦ Ⓣ Ⓕ ● ●

Muscle Group Focus ___________ Weight ________ Date/Time ___________

Stretch ◯   Warm-Up _________________________________

Strength Training

Exercise		Set 1	Set 2	Set 3	Set 4	Set 5	Set 6
	Reps						
	Weight						
	Reps						
	Weight						
	Reps						
	Weight						
	Reps						
	Weight						
	Reps						
	Weight						
	Reps						
	Weight						
	Reps						
	Weight						
	Reps						
	Weight						
	Reps						
	Weight						

Cardio

Exercise	Calories	Distance	Time

Water Intake ___________

Cooldown ___________

Feeling ☆☆☆☆☆

Notes

Today's Goal __________ Ⓜ Ⓣ Ⓦ Ⓣ Ⓕ ⬤S ⬤S

Muscle Group Focus __________   Weight __________   Date/Time __________

Stretch ◯   Warm-Up __________

Strength Training

Exercise		Set 1	Set 2	Set 3	Set 4	Set 5	Set 6
	Reps						
	Weight						
	Reps						
	Weight						
	Reps						
	Weight						
	Reps						
	Weight						
	Reps						
	Weight						
	Reps						
	Weight						
	Reps						
	Weight						
	Reps						
	Weight						
	Reps						
	Weight						

Cardio

Exercise	Calories	Distance	Time

Water Intake __________

Cooldown __________

Feeling ☆ ☆ ☆ ☆ ☆

Notes

Today's Goal _____________ Ⓜ Ⓣ Ⓦ Ⓣ Ⓕ ⬤S ⬤S

Muscle Group Focus __________   Weight ________   Date/Time __________

Stretch ◯   Warm-Up _______________________________________

Strength Training

Exercise		Set 1	Set 2	Set 3	Set 4	Set 5	Set 6
	Reps						
	Weight						
	Reps						
	Weight						
	Reps						
	Weight						
	Reps						
	Weight						
	Reps						
	Weight						
	Reps						
	Weight						
	Reps						
	Weight						
	Reps						
	Weight						
	Reps						
	Weight						

Cardio

Exercise	Calories	Distance	Time

Water Intake _______________________

Cooldown _______________________

Feeling ☆ ☆ ☆ ☆ ☆

Notes

Today's Goal _____________ Ⓜ Ⓣ Ⓦ Ⓣ Ⓕ ⬤S ⬤S

Muscle Group Focus __________   Weight ________   Date/Time __________

Stretch ◯   Warm-Up _______________________________

Strength Training

Exercise		Set 1	Set 2	Set 3	Set 4	Set 5	Set 6
	Reps						
	Weight						
	Reps						
	Weight						
	Reps						
	Weight						
	Reps						
	Weight						
	Reps						
	Weight						
	Reps						
	Weight						
	Reps						
	Weight						
	Reps						
	Weight						
	Reps						
	Weight						
	Reps						
	Weight						

Cardio

Exercise	Calories	Distance	Time

Water Intake _______________

Cooldown _______________

Feeling ☆ ☆ ☆ ☆ ☆

Notes

Today's Goal _______   Ⓜ Ⓣ Ⓦ Ⓣ Ⓕ ⬤S ⬤S

Muscle Group Focus _______   Weight _______   Date/Time _______

Stretch ◯   Warm-Up _______________________________

Strength Training

Exercise		Set 1	Set 2	Set 3	Set 4	Set 5	Set 6
	Reps						
	Weight						
	Reps						
	Weight						
	Reps						
	Weight						
	Reps						
	Weight						
	Reps						
	Weight						
	Reps						
	Weight						
	Reps						
	Weight						
	Reps						
	Weight						
	Reps						
	Weight						
	Reps						
	Weight						

Cardio

Exercise	Calories	Distance	Time

Water Intake _______________

Cooldown _______________

Feeling ☆ ☆ ☆ ☆ ☆

Notes

Today's Goal ____________   (M) (T) (W) (T) (F) (S) (S)

Muscle Group Focus ____________   Weight ________   Date/Time ____________

Stretch ◯   Warm-Up ____________________________

Strength Training

Exercise		Set 1	Set 2	Set 3	Set 4	Set 5	Set 6
	Reps						
	Weight						
	Reps						
	Weight						
	Reps						
	Weight						
	Reps						
	Weight						
	Reps						
	Weight						
	Reps						
	Weight						
	Reps						
	Weight						
	Reps						
	Weight						

Cardio

Exercise	Calories	Distance	Time

Water Intake ____________________

Cooldown ____________________

Feeling ☆ ☆ ☆ ☆ ☆

Notes

Today's Goal ___________ Ⓜ Ⓣ Ⓦ Ⓣ Ⓕ ⬤S ⬤S

Muscle Group Focus __________   Weight ________   Date/Time __________

Stretch ◯   Warm-Up ____

Strength Training

Exercise		Set 1	Set 2	Set 3	Set 4	Set 5	Set 6
	Reps						
	Weight						
	Reps						
	Weight						
	Reps						
	Weight						
	Reps						
	Weight						
	Reps						
	Weight						
	Reps						
	Weight						
	Reps						
	Weight						
	Reps						
	Weight						
	Reps						
	Weight						

Cardio

Exercise	Calories	Distance	Time

Water Intake ________________

Cooldown ________________

Feeling ☆ ☆ ☆ ☆ ☆

Notes

Today's Goal _____________ Ⓜ Ⓣ Ⓦ Ⓣ Ⓕ Ⓢ Ⓢ

Muscle Group Focus __________   Weight ________   Date/Time __________

Stretch ◯   Warm-Up _______________________________

Strength Training

Exercise		Set 1	Set 2	Set 3	Set 4	Set 5	Set 6
	Reps						
	Weight						
	Reps						
	Weight						
	Reps						
	Weight						
	Reps						
	Weight						
	Reps						
	Weight						
	Reps						
	Weight						
	Reps						
	Weight						
	Reps						
	Weight						
	Reps						
	Weight						
	Reps						
	Weight						

Cardio

Exercise	Calories	Distance	Time

Water Intake _______________

Cooldown _______________

Feeling ☆ ☆ ☆ ☆ ☆

Notes

Today's Goal _____________ Ⓜ Ⓣ Ⓦ Ⓣ Ⓕ ⬤S ⬤S

Muscle Group Focus __________   Weight ________   Date/Time __________

Stretch ◯   Warm-Up _________________________________

Strength Training

Exercise		Set 1	Set 2	Set 3	Set 4	Set 5	Set 6
	Reps						
	Weight						
	Reps						
	Weight						
	Reps						
	Weight						
	Reps						
	Weight						
	Reps						
	Weight						
	Reps						
	Weight						
	Reps						
	Weight						
	Reps						
	Weight						
	Reps						
	Weight						

Cardio

Exercise	Calories	Distance	Time

Water Intake _________________

Cooldown _________________

Feeling ☆ ☆ ☆ ☆ ☆

Notes

Today's Goal ________________   (M) (T) (W) (T) (F) (S) (S)

Muscle Group Focus __________   Weight ________   Date/Time __________

Stretch ◯   Warm-Up ________________________________

Strength Training

Exercise		Set 1	Set 2	Set 3	Set 4	Set 5	Set 6
	Reps						
	Weight						
	Reps						
	Weight						
	Reps						
	Weight						
	Reps						
	Weight						
	Reps						
	Weight						
	Reps						
	Weight						
	Reps						
	Weight						
	Reps						
	Weight						
	Reps						
	Weight						

Cardio

Exercise	Calories	Distance	Time

Water Intake ________________

Cooldown ________________

Feeling ☆ ☆ ☆ ☆ ☆

Notes

Today's Goal ______________   (M) (T) (W) (T) (F) (S) (S)

Muscle Group Focus ___________   Weight ________   Date/Time ___________

Stretch ◯   Warm-Up ____

Strength Training

Exercise		Set 1	Set 2	Set 3	Set 4	Set 5	Set 6
	Reps						
	Weight						
	Reps						
	Weight						
	Reps						
	Weight						
	Reps						
	Weight						
	Reps						
	Weight						
	Reps						
	Weight						
	Reps						
	Weight						
	Reps						
	Weight						

Cardio

Exercise	Calories	Distance	Time

Water Intake ________________

Cooldown ________________

Feeling ☆ ☆ ☆ ☆ ☆

Notes

Today's Goal _____________ M T W T F **S** **S**

Muscle Group Focus ___________ Weight ________ Date/Time ___________

Stretch ◯ Warm-Up ___________________________

Strength Training

Exercise		Set 1	Set 2	Set 3	Set 4	Set 5	Set 6
	Reps						
	Weight						
	Reps						
	Weight						
	Reps						
	Weight						
	Reps						
	Weight						
	Reps						
	Weight						
	Reps						
	Weight						
	Reps						
	Weight						
	Reps						
	Weight						
	Reps						
	Weight						

Cardio

Exercise	Calories	Distance	Time

Water Intake ___________________

Cooldown ___________________

Feeling ☆ ☆ ☆ ☆ ☆

Notes

Today's Goal

(M) (T) (W) (T) (F) (S) (S)

Muscle Group Focus ___________ Weight _________ Date/Time ___________

Stretch ◯ Warm-Up _________________________________

Strength Training

Exercise		Set 1	Set 2	Set 3	Set 4	Set 5	Set 6
	Reps						
	Weight						
	Reps						
	Weight						
	Reps						
	Weight						
	Reps						
	Weight						
	Reps						
	Weight						
	Reps						
	Weight						
	Reps						
	Weight						
	Reps						
	Weight						
	Reps						
	Weight						

Cardio

Exercise	Calories	Distance	Time

Water Intake _________________________

Cooldown _________________________

Feeling ☆ ☆ ☆ ☆ ☆

Notes

Today's Goal ______________ Ⓜ Ⓣ Ⓦ Ⓣ Ⓕ Ⓢ Ⓢ

Muscle Group Focus __________ Weight ________ Date/Time __________

Stretch ◯ Warm-Up ____________________________

Strength Training

Exercise		Set 1	Set 2	Set 3	Set 4	Set 5	Set 6
	Reps						
	Weight						
	Reps						
	Weight						
	Reps						
	Weight						
	Reps						
	Weight						
	Reps						
	Weight						
	Reps						
	Weight						
	Reps						
	Weight						
	Reps						
	Weight						
	Reps						
	Weight						

Cardio

Exercise	Calories	Distance	Time

Water Intake ____________________

Cooldown ____________________

Feeling ☆ ☆ ☆ ☆ ☆

Notes

Today's Goal _______________   (M) (T) (W) (T) (F) (S) (S)

Muscle Group Focus _______   Weight _______   Date/Time _______

Stretch ◯   Warm-Up _______________________________

Strength Training

Exercise		Set 1	Set 2	Set 3	Set 4	Set 5	Set 6
	Reps						
	Weight						
	Reps						
	Weight						
	Reps						
	Weight						
	Reps						
	Weight						
	Reps						
	Weight						
	Reps						
	Weight						
	Reps						
	Weight						
	Reps						
	Weight						
	Reps						
	Weight						
	Reps						
	Weight						

Cardio

Exercise	Calories	Distance	Time

Water Intake _______________________

Cooldown _______________________

Feeling ☆ ☆ ☆ ☆ ☆

Notes

Today's Goal ___________ (M) (T) (W) (T) (F) **(S)** **(S)**

Muscle Group Focus ___________   Weight _________   Date/Time ___________

Stretch ◯   Warm-Up ___________

Strength Training

Exercise		Set 1	Set 2	Set 3	Set 4	Set 5	Set 6
	Reps						
	Weight						
	Reps						
	Weight						
	Reps						
	Weight						
	Reps						
	Weight						
	Reps						
	Weight						
	Reps						
	Weight						
	Reps						
	Weight						
	Reps						
	Weight						
	Reps						
	Weight						
	Reps						
	Weight						

Cardio

Exercise	Calories	Distance	Time

Water Intake ___________

Cooldown ___________

Feeling ☆ ☆ ☆ ☆ ☆

Notes

Today's Goal _____________   (M) (T) (W) (T) (F) (S) (S)

Muscle Group Focus _________   Weight _______   Date/Time _________

Stretch ◯   Warm-Up ____

Strength Training

Exercise		Set 1	Set 2	Set 3	Set 4	Set 5	Set 6
	Reps						
	Weight						
	Reps						
	Weight						
	Reps						
	Weight						
	Reps						
	Weight						
	Reps						
	Weight						
	Reps						
	Weight						
	Reps						
	Weight						
	Reps						
	Weight						
	Reps						
	Weight						

Cardio

Exercise	Calories	Distance	Time

Water Intake _________________

Cooldown _________________

Feeling ☆ ☆ ☆ ☆ ☆

Notes

Today's Goal ⓂⓉⓌⓉⒻ ● ●

Muscle Group Focus __________   Weight ________   Date/Time __________

Stretch ◯   Warm-Up __________________________________

Strength Training

Exercise		Set 1	Set 2	Set 3	Set 4	Set 5	Set 6
	Reps						
	Weight						
	Reps						
	Weight						
	Reps						
	Weight						
	Reps						
	Weight						
	Reps						
	Weight						
	Reps						
	Weight						
	Reps						
	Weight						
	Reps						
	Weight						
	Reps						
	Weight						

Cardio

Exercise	Calories	Distance	Time

Water Intake __________________

Cooldown __________________

Feeling ☆ ☆ ☆ ☆ ☆

Notes

Today's Goal _____________   Ⓜ Ⓣ Ⓦ Ⓣ Ⓕ ⬤S ⬤S

Muscle Group Focus __________   Weight ________   Date/Time __________

Stretch ◯   Warm-Up _________________________________

Strength Training

Exercise		Set 1	Set 2	Set 3	Set 4	Set 5	Set 6
	Reps						
	Weight						
	Reps						
	Weight						
	Reps						
	Weight						
	Reps						
	Weight						
	Reps						
	Weight						
	Reps						
	Weight						
	Reps						
	Weight						
	Reps						
	Weight						
	Reps						
	Weight						

Cardio

Exercise	Calories	Distance	Time

Water Intake _________________

Cooldown _________________

Feeling ☆ ☆ ☆ ☆ ☆

Notes

Today's Goal ___________ (M) (T) (W) (T) (F) (S) (S)

Muscle Group Focus ___________   Weight _________   Date/Time ___________

Stretch ◯   Warm-Up _________________________________

Strength Training

Exercise		Set 1	Set 2	Set 3	Set 4	Set 5	Set 6
	Reps						
	Weight						
	Reps						
	Weight						
	Reps						
	Weight						
	Reps						
	Weight						
	Reps						
	Weight						
	Reps						
	Weight						
	Reps						
	Weight						
	Reps						
	Weight						
	Reps						
	Weight						
	Reps						
	Weight						

Cardio

Exercise	Calories	Distance	Time

Water Intake ___________

Cooldown ___________

Feeling ☆ ☆ ☆ ☆ ☆

Notes

Today's Goal _____________   Ⓜ Ⓣ Ⓦ Ⓣ Ⓕ ⬤S ⬤S

Muscle Group Focus __________   Weight _______   Date/Time __________

Stretch ◯   Warm-Up _______________________________

Strength Training

Exercise		Set 1	Set 2	Set 3	Set 4	Set 5	Set 6
	Reps						
	Weight						
	Reps						
	Weight						
	Reps						
	Weight						
	Reps						
	Weight						
	Reps						
	Weight						
	Reps						
	Weight						
	Reps						
	Weight						
	Reps						
	Weight						
	Reps						
	Weight						
	Reps						
	Weight						

Cardio

Exercise	Calories	Distance	Time

Water Intake _______________

Cooldown _______________

Feeling ☆ ☆ ☆ ☆ ☆

Notes

Today's Goal ____________ Ⓜ Ⓣ Ⓦ Ⓣ Ⓕ Ⓢ Ⓢ

Muscle Group Focus ___________ Weight _________ Date/Time ___________

Stretch ◯   Warm-Up ________________________________

Strength Training

Exercise		Set 1	Set 2	Set 3	Set 4	Set 5	Set 6
	Reps						
	Weight						
	Reps						
	Weight						
	Reps						
	Weight						
	Reps						
	Weight						
	Reps						
	Weight						
	Reps						
	Weight						
	Reps						
	Weight						
	Reps						
	Weight						
	Reps						
	Weight						

Cardio

Exercise	Calories	Distance	Time

Water Intake ________________

Cooldown ________________

Feeling ☆ ☆ ☆ ☆ ☆

Notes

Today's Goal   _______________   (M) (T) (W) (T) (F) (S) (S)

Muscle Group Focus ___________   Weight _________   Date/Time _____________

Stretch ◯   Warm-Up ____

Strength Training

Exercise		Set 1	Set 2	Set 3	Set 4	Set 5	Set 6
	Reps						
	Weight						
	Reps						
	Weight						
	Reps						
	Weight						
	Reps						
	Weight						
	Reps						
	Weight						
	Reps						
	Weight						
	Reps						
	Weight						
	Reps						
	Weight						
	Reps						
	Weight						
	Reps						
	Weight						

Cardio

Exercise	Calories	Distance	Time

Water Intake ___________________

Cooldown ___________________

Feeling ☆ ☆ ☆ ☆ ☆

Notes

Today's Goal _____________   Ⓜ Ⓣ Ⓦ Ⓣ Ⓕ ⬤S ⬤S

Muscle Group Focus ___________   Weight ________   Date/Time ____________

Stretch ◯   Warm-Up ________________________________

Strength Training

Exercise		Set 1	Set 2	Set 3	Set 4	Set 5	Set 6
	Reps						
	Weight						
	Reps						
	Weight						
	Reps						
	Weight						
	Reps						
	Weight						
	Reps						
	Weight						
	Reps						
	Weight						
	Reps						
	Weight						
	Reps						
	Weight						
	Reps						
	Weight						

Cardio

Exercise	Calories	Distance	Time

Water Intake ________________

Cooldown ________________

Feeling ☆ ☆ ☆ ☆ ☆

Notes

Today's Goal ______________   M T W T F S S

Muscle Group Focus __________   Weight ________   Date/Time __________

Stretch ◯   Warm-Up ________________________________

Strength Training

Exercise		Set 1	Set 2	Set 3	Set 4	Set 5	Set 6
	Reps						
	Weight						
	Reps						
	Weight						
	Reps						
	Weight						
	Reps						
	Weight						
	Reps						
	Weight						
	Reps						
	Weight						
	Reps						
	Weight						
	Reps						
	Weight						

Cardio

Exercise	Calories	Distance	Time

Water Intake ________________

Cooldown ________________

Feeling ☆ ☆ ☆ ☆ ☆

Notes

Today's Goal ______________   Ⓜ Ⓣ Ⓦ Ⓣ Ⓕ ⬤S ⬤S

Muscle Group Focus ___________   Weight ________   Date/Time ___________

Stretch ◯   Warm-Up ___________________________

Strength Training

Exercise		Set 1	Set 2	Set 3	Set 4	Set 5	Set 6
	Reps						
	Weight						
	Reps						
	Weight						
	Reps						
	Weight						
	Reps						
	Weight						
	Reps						
	Weight						
	Reps						
	Weight						
	Reps						
	Weight						
	Reps						
	Weight						
	Reps						
	Weight						

Cardio

Exercise	Calories	Distance	Time

Water Intake ___________________

Cooldown ___________________

Feeling ☆ ☆ ☆ ☆ ☆

Notes

Today's Goal ___________ Ⓜ Ⓣ Ⓦ Ⓣ Ⓕ ⬤S ⬤S

Muscle Group Focus __________   Weight ________   Date/Time __________

Stretch ◯   Warm-Up ________________________________

Strength Training

Exercise		Set 1	Set 2	Set 3	Set 4	Set 5	Set 6
	Reps						
	Weight						
	Reps						
	Weight						
	Reps						
	Weight						
	Reps						
	Weight						
	Reps						
	Weight						
	Reps						
	Weight						
	Reps						
	Weight						
	Reps						
	Weight						
	Reps						
	Weight						
	Reps						
	Weight						

Cardio

Exercise	Calories	Distance	Time

Water Intake ________________

Cooldown ________________

Feeling ☆ ☆ ☆ ☆ ☆

Notes

Today's Goal __________ Ⓜ Ⓣ Ⓦ Ⓣ Ⓕ ⬤S ⬤S

Muscle Group Focus __________ Weight __________ Date/Time __________

Stretch ◯   Warm-Up __________

Strength Training

Exercise		Set 1	Set 2	Set 3	Set 4	Set 5	Set 6
	Reps						
	Weight						
	Reps						
	Weight						
	Reps						
	Weight						
	Reps						
	Weight						
	Reps						
	Weight						
	Reps						
	Weight						
	Reps						
	Weight						
	Reps						
	Weight						
	Reps						
	Weight						

Cardio

Exercise	Calories	Distance	Time

Water Intake __________

Cooldown __________

Feeling ☆ ☆ ☆ ☆ ☆

Notes

Today's Goal ___________   (M) (T) (W) (T) (F) (S) (S)

Muscle Group Focus __________   Weight ________   Date/Time __________

Stretch ◯   Warm-Up ________________________________

Strength Training

Exercise		Set 1	Set 2	Set 3	Set 4	Set 5	Set 6
	Reps						
	Weight						
	Reps						
	Weight						
	Reps						
	Weight						
	Reps						
	Weight						
	Reps						
	Weight						
	Reps						
	Weight						
	Reps						
	Weight						
	Reps						
	Weight						
	Reps						
	Weight						

Cardio

Exercise	Calories	Distance	Time

Water Intake ________________

Cooldown ____________

Feeling ☆ ☆ ☆ ☆ ☆

Notes

Today's Goal ___________ Ⓜ Ⓣ Ⓦ Ⓣ Ⓕ ● ●

Muscle Group Focus ___________   Weight _______   Date/Time ___________

Stretch ◯   Warm-Up ___________________________________

Strength Training

Exercise		Set 1	Set 2	Set 3	Set 4	Set 5	Set 6
	Reps						
	Weight						
	Reps						
	Weight						
	Reps						
	Weight						
	Reps						
	Weight						
	Reps						
	Weight						
	Reps						
	Weight						
	Reps						
	Weight						
	Reps						
	Weight						
	Reps						
	Weight						
	Reps						
	Weight						

Cardio

Exercise	Calories	Distance	Time

Water Intake ___________________

Cooldown ___________________

Feeling ☆ ☆ ☆ ☆ ☆

Notes

Today's Goal _____________ Ⓜ Ⓣ Ⓦ Ⓣ Ⓕ ● ●

Muscle Group Focus __________   Weight ________   Date/Time ____________

Stretch ◯   Warm-Up ________________________________

Strength Training

Exercise		Set 1	Set 2	Set 3	Set 4	Set 5	Set 6
	Reps						
	Weight						
	Reps						
	Weight						
	Reps						
	Weight						
	Reps						
	Weight						
	Reps						
	Weight						
	Reps						
	Weight						
	Reps						
	Weight						
	Reps						
	Weight						
	Reps						
	Weight						
	Reps						
	Weight						

Cardio

Exercise	Calories	Distance	Time

Water Intake _________________

Cooldown _________________

Feeling ☆ ☆ ☆ ☆ ☆

Notes

Today's Goal ______________   (M) (T) (W) (T) (F) (S) (S)

Muscle Group Focus ___________   Weight ________   Date/Time __________

Stretch ◯   Warm-Up ________________________

Strength Training

Exercise		Set 1	Set 2	Set 3	Set 4	Set 5	Set 6
	Reps						
	Weight						
	Reps						
	Weight						
	Reps						
	Weight						
	Reps						
	Weight						
	Reps						
	Weight						
	Reps						
	Weight						
	Reps						
	Weight						
	Reps						
	Weight						
	Reps						
	Weight						
	Reps						
	Weight						

Cardio

Exercise	Calories	Distance	Time

Water Intake ________________

Cooldown ________________

Feeling ☆ ☆ ☆ ☆ ☆

Notes

Today's Goal ______________   (M) (T) (W) (T) (F) (S) (S)

Muscle Group Focus __________   Weight ________   Date/Time __________

Stretch ◯   Warm-Up _______________________________________

Strength Training

Exercise		Set 1	Set 2	Set 3	Set 4	Set 5	Set 6
	Reps						
	Weight						
	Reps						
	Weight						
	Reps						
	Weight						
	Reps						
	Weight						
	Reps						
	Weight						
	Reps						
	Weight						
	Reps						
	Weight						
	Reps						
	Weight						

Cardio

Exercise	Calories	Distance	Time

Water Intake _______________

Cooldown _______________

Feeling ☆ ☆ ☆ ☆ ☆

Notes

Today's Goal ____________ (M) (T) (W) (T) (F) (S) (S)

Muscle Group Focus __________   Weight ________   Date/Time __________

Stretch ◯   Warm-Up ________________________________

Strength Training

Exercise		Set 1	Set 2	Set 3	Set 4	Set 5	Set 6
	Reps						
	Weight						
	Reps						
	Weight						
	Reps						
	Weight						
	Reps						
	Weight						
	Reps						
	Weight						
	Reps						
	Weight						
	Reps						
	Weight						
	Reps						
	Weight						
	Reps						
	Weight						
	Reps						
	Weight						

Cardio

Exercise	Calories	Distance	Time

Water Intake ________________

Cooldown ________________

Feeling ☆ ☆ ☆ ☆ ☆

Notes

Today's Goal _____________   Ⓜ Ⓣ Ⓦ Ⓣ Ⓕ ⬤S ⬤S

Muscle Group Focus _________   Weight _______   Date/Time _________

Stretch ◯   Warm-Up _______________________________

Strength Training

Exercise		Set 1	Set 2	Set 3	Set 4	Set 5	Set 6
	Reps						
	Weight						
	Reps						
	Weight						
	Reps						
	Weight						
	Reps						
	Weight						
	Reps						
	Weight						
	Reps						
	Weight						
	Reps						
	Weight						
	Reps						
	Weight						
	Reps						
	Weight						

Cardio

Exercise	Calories	Distance	Time

Water Intake _______________

Cooldown _______________

Feeling ☆ ☆ ☆ ☆ ☆

Notes

Today's Goal ____________   Ⓜ Ⓣ Ⓦ Ⓣ Ⓕ Ⓢ Ⓢ

Muscle Group Focus __________   Weight ________   Date/Time __________

Stretch ◯   Warm-Up ________________________________

Strength Training

Exercise		Set 1	Set 2	Set 3	Set 4	Set 5	Set 6
	Reps						
	Weight						
	Reps						
	Weight						
	Reps						
	Weight						
	Reps						
	Weight						
	Reps						
	Weight						
	Reps						
	Weight						
	Reps						
	Weight						
	Reps						
	Weight						
	Reps						
	Weight						
	Reps						
	Weight						

Cardio

Exercise	Calories	Distance	Time

Water Intake ________________

Cooldown ________________

Feeling ☆ ☆ ☆ ☆ ☆

Notes

Today's Goal _______________ Ⓜ Ⓣ Ⓦ Ⓣ Ⓕ Ⓢ Ⓢ

Muscle Group Focus __________ Weight ________ Date/Time __________

Stretch ◯   Warm-Up _______________________________

Strength Training

Exercise		Set 1	Set 2	Set 3	Set 4	Set 5	Set 6
	Reps						
	Weight						
	Reps						
	Weight						
	Reps						
	Weight						
	Reps						
	Weight						
	Reps						
	Weight						
	Reps						
	Weight						
	Reps						
	Weight						
	Reps						
	Weight						
	Reps						
	Weight						

Cardio

Exercise	Calories	Distance	Time

Water Intake _______________

Cooldown _______________

Feeling ☆ ☆ ☆ ☆ ☆

Notes

Strength Training

Exercise		Set 1	Set 2	Set 3	Set 4	Set 5	Set 6
	Reps						
	Weight						
	Reps						
	Weight						
	Reps						
	Weight						
	Reps						
	Weight						
	Reps						
	Weight						
	Reps						
	Weight						
	Reps						
	Weight						
	Reps						
	Weight						

Cardio

Exercise	Calories	Distance	Time

Water Intake ______

Cooldown ______

Feeling ☆ ☆ ☆ ☆ ☆

Notes

Today's Goal ____________ Ⓜ Ⓣ Ⓦ Ⓣ Ⓕ ● ●

Muscle Group Focus __________ Weight ________ Date/Time __________

Stretch ◯   Warm-Up ________________________________

Strength Training

Exercise		Set 1	Set 2	Set 3	Set 4	Set 5	Set 6
	Reps						
	Weight						
	Reps						
	Weight						
	Reps						
	Weight						
	Reps						
	Weight						
	Reps						
	Weight						
	Reps						
	Weight						
	Reps						
	Weight						
	Reps						
	Weight						
	Reps						
	Weight						
	Reps						
	Weight						

Cardio

Exercise	Calories	Distance	Time

Water Intake ________________

Cooldown ________________

Feeling ☆ ☆ ☆ ☆ ☆

Notes

Today's Goal ________________ (M) (T) (W) (T) (F) (S) (S)

Muscle Group Focus __________   Weight ________   Date/Time __________

Stretch ◯   Warm-Up ________________________________

Strength Training

Exercise		Set 1	Set 2	Set 3	Set 4	Set 5	Set 6
	Reps						
	Weight						
	Reps						
	Weight						
	Reps						
	Weight						
	Reps						
	Weight						
	Reps						
	Weight						
	Reps						
	Weight						
	Reps						
	Weight						
	Reps						
	Weight						
	Reps						
	Weight						
	Reps						
	Weight						

Cardio

Exercise	Calories	Distance	Time

Water Intake ________________

Cooldown ________________

Feeling ☆ ☆ ☆ ☆ ☆

Notes

Today's Goal _______________   (M) (T) (W) (T) (F) (S) (S)

Muscle Group Focus __________   Weight ________   Date/Time ___________

Stretch ◯   Warm-Up ____________________________________

Strength Training

Exercise		Set 1	Set 2	Set 3	Set 4	Set 5	Set 6
	Reps						
	Weight						
	Reps						
	Weight						
	Reps						
	Weight						
	Reps						
	Weight						
	Reps						
	Weight						
	Reps						
	Weight						
	Reps						
	Weight						
	Reps						
	Weight						
	Reps						
	Weight						
	Reps						
	Weight						

Cardio

Exercise	Calories	Distance	Time

Water Intake ____________________

Cooldown ____________________

Feeling ☆ ☆ ☆ ☆ ☆

Notes

Today's Goal ___________ (M) (T) (W) (T) (F) ● S ● S

Muscle Group Focus ___________   Weight _________   Date/Time ___________

Stretch ◯   Warm-Up ____

Strength Training

Exercise		Set 1	Set 2	Set 3	Set 4	Set 5	Set 6
	Reps						
	Weight						
	Reps						
	Weight						
	Reps						
	Weight						
	Reps						
	Weight						
	Reps						
	Weight						
	Reps						
	Weight						
	Reps						
	Weight						
	Reps						
	Weight						
	Reps						
	Weight						
	Reps						
	Weight						

Cardio

Exercise	Calories	Distance	Time

Water Intake ___________________

Cooldown ___________________

Feeling ☆ ☆ ☆ ☆ ☆

Notes

Today's Goal ___________ Ⓜ Ⓣ Ⓦ Ⓣ Ⓕ ⬤S ⬤S

Muscle Group Focus __________ Weight ________ Date/Time __________

Stretch ◯ Warm-Up _______________________________

Strength Training

Exercise		Set 1	Set 2	Set 3	Set 4	Set 5	Set 6
	Reps						
	Weight						
	Reps						
	Weight						
	Reps						
	Weight						
	Reps						
	Weight						
	Reps						
	Weight						
	Reps						
	Weight						
	Reps						
	Weight						
	Reps						
	Weight						
	Reps						
	Weight						
	Reps						
	Weight						

Cardio

Exercise	Calories	Distance	Time

Water Intake _______________

Cooldown _______________

Feeling ☆ ☆ ☆ ☆ ☆

Notes

Today's Goal ________   Ⓜ Ⓣ Ⓦ Ⓣ Ⓕ Ⓢ Ⓢ

Muscle Group Focus ________   Weight ________   Date/Time ________

Stretch ◯   Warm-Up ________

Strength Training

Exercise		Set 1	Set 2	Set 3	Set 4	Set 5	Set 6
	Reps						
	Weight						
	Reps						
	Weight						
	Reps						
	Weight						
	Reps						
	Weight						
	Reps						
	Weight						
	Reps						
	Weight						
	Reps						
	Weight						
	Reps						
	Weight						
	Reps						
	Weight						
	Reps						
	Weight						

Cardio

Exercise	Calories	Distance	Time

Water Intake ________

Cooldown ________

Feeling ☆ ☆ ☆ ☆ ☆

Notes

Today's Goal _____________ Ⓜ Ⓣ Ⓦ Ⓣ Ⓕ Ⓢ Ⓢ

Muscle Group Focus __________   Weight ________   Date/Time ___________

Stretch ◯   Warm-Up ________________________________

Strength Training

Exercise		Set 1	Set 2	Set 3	Set 4	Set 5	Set 6
	Reps						
	Weight						
	Reps						
	Weight						
	Reps						
	Weight						
	Reps						
	Weight						
	Reps						
	Weight						
	Reps						
	Weight						
	Reps						
	Weight						
	Reps						
	Weight						

Cardio

Exercise	Calories	Distance	Time

Water Intake ___________________

Cooldown ___________________

Feeling ☆ ☆ ☆ ☆ ☆

Notes

Today's Goal ___________ Ⓜ Ⓣ Ⓦ Ⓣ Ⓕ ⚫S ⚫S

Muscle Group Focus ___________ Weight ________ Date/Time ___________

Stretch ◯   Warm-Up ____

Strength Training

Exercise		Set 1	Set 2	Set 3	Set 4	Set 5	Set 6
	Reps						
	Weight						
	Reps						
	Weight						
	Reps						
	Weight						
	Reps						
	Weight						
	Reps						
	Weight						
	Reps						
	Weight						
	Reps						
	Weight						
	Reps						
	Weight						
	Reps						
	Weight						

Cardio

Exercise	Calories	Distance	Time

Water Intake ___________________

Cooldown ___________________

Feeling ☆ ☆ ☆ ☆ ☆

Notes

Today's Goal ___________ Ⓜ Ⓣ Ⓦ Ⓣ Ⓕ ⬤S ⬤S

Muscle Group Focus __________ Weight ________ Date/Time __________

Stretch ◯   Warm-Up ____________________________________

Strength Training

Exercise		Set 1	Set 2	Set 3	Set 4	Set 5	Set 6
	Reps						
	Weight						
	Reps						
	Weight						
	Reps						
	Weight						
	Reps						
	Weight						
	Reps						
	Weight						
	Reps						
	Weight						
	Reps						
	Weight						
	Reps						
	Weight						
	Reps						
	Weight						
	Reps						
	Weight						

Cardio

Exercise	Calories	Distance	Time

Water Intake ____________________

Cooldown ____________________

Feeling ☆ ☆ ☆ ☆ ☆

Notes

Today's Goal ____________   Ⓜ Ⓣ Ⓦ Ⓣ Ⓕ ⬤S ⬤S

Muscle Group Focus __________   Weight ________   Date/Time __________

Stretch ◯   Warm-Up ________________________

Strength Training

Exercise		Set 1	Set 2	Set 3	Set 4	Set 5	Set 6
	Reps						
	Weight						
	Reps						
	Weight						
	Reps						
	Weight						
	Reps						
	Weight						
	Reps						
	Weight						
	Reps						
	Weight						
	Reps						
	Weight						
	Reps						
	Weight						
	Reps						
	Weight						
	Reps						
	Weight						

Cardio

Exercise	Calories	Distance	Time

Water Intake ________________

Cooldown ________________

Feeling ☆ ☆ ☆ ☆ ☆

Notes

Today's Goal ____________ Ⓜ Ⓣ Ⓦ Ⓣ Ⓕ ⬤S ⬤S

Muscle Group Focus ___________ Weight ________ Date/Time ___________

Stretch ◯   Warm-Up ________________________________

Strength Training

Exercise		Set 1	Set 2	Set 3	Set 4	Set 5	Set 6
	Reps						
	Weight						
	Reps						
	Weight						
	Reps						
	Weight						
	Reps						
	Weight						
	Reps						
	Weight						
	Reps						
	Weight						
	Reps						
	Weight						
	Reps						
	Weight						
	Reps						
	Weight						
	Reps						
	Weight						

Cardio

Exercise	Calories	Distance	Time

Water Intake ___________

Cooldown ___________

Feeling ☆ ☆ ☆ ☆ ☆

Notes

Today's Goal _______________ Ⓜ Ⓣ Ⓦ Ⓣ Ⓕ ⚫S ⚫S

Muscle Group Focus _____________ Weight _________ Date/Time _____________

Stretch ◯   Warm-Up _______________________________

Strength Training

Exercise		Set 1	Set 2	Set 3	Set 4	Set 5	Set 6
	Reps						
	Weight						
	Reps						
	Weight						
	Reps						
	Weight						
	Reps						
	Weight						
	Reps						
	Weight						
	Reps						
	Weight						
	Reps						
	Weight						
	Reps						
	Weight						
	Reps						
	Weight						

Cardio

Exercise	Calories	Distance	Time

Water Intake _______________

Cooldown _______________

Feeling ☆ ☆ ☆ ☆ ☆

Notes

Today's Goal _____________ Ⓜ Ⓣ Ⓦ Ⓣ Ⓕ ⚫S ⚫S

Muscle Group Focus __________ Weight ________ Date/Time __________

Stretch ◯   Warm-Up ________________________________

Strength Training

Exercise		Set 1	Set 2	Set 3	Set 4	Set 5	Set 6
	Reps						
	Weight						
	Reps						
	Weight						
	Reps						
	Weight						
	Reps						
	Weight						
	Reps						
	Weight						
	Reps						
	Weight						
	Reps						
	Weight						
	Reps						
	Weight						
	Reps						
	Weight						
	Reps						
	Weight						

Cardio

Exercise	Calories	Distance	Time

Water Intake ________________

Cooldown ________________

Feeling ☆ ☆ ☆ ☆ ☆

Notes

Today's Goal ___________   (M) (T) (W) (T) (F) (S) (S)

Muscle Group Focus __________   Weight ________   Date/Time __________

Stretch ◯   Warm-Up ________________________

Strength Training

Exercise		Set 1	Set 2	Set 3	Set 4	Set 5	Set 6
	Reps						
	Weight						
	Reps						
	Weight						
	Reps						
	Weight						
	Reps						
	Weight						
	Reps						
	Weight						
	Reps						
	Weight						
	Reps						
	Weight						
	Reps						
	Weight						
	Reps						
	Weight						
	Reps						
	Weight						

Cardio

Exercise	Calories	Distance	Time

Water Intake ________________

Cooldown ________________

Feeling ☆ ☆ ☆ ☆ ☆

Notes

Today's Goal ___________ (M) (T) (W) (T) (F) (S) (S)

Muscle Group Focus ___________ Weight _______ Date/Time _________

Stretch ◯ Warm-Up _________________________________

Strength Training

Exercise		Set 1	Set 2	Set 3	Set 4	Set 5	Set 6
	Reps						
	Weight						
	Reps						
	Weight						
	Reps						
	Weight						
	Reps						
	Weight						
	Reps						
	Weight						
	Reps						
	Weight						
	Reps						
	Weight						
	Reps						
	Weight						
	Reps						
	Weight						

Cardio

Exercise	Calories	Distance	Time

Water Intake _________________

Cooldown _________________

Feeling ☆ ☆ ☆ ☆ ☆

Notes

Today's Goal _______________   (M) (T) (W) (T) (F) (S) (S)

Muscle Group Focus ___________   Weight _________   Date/Time _____________

Stretch ◯   Warm-Up ____

Strength Training

Exercise		Set 1	Set 2	Set 3	Set 4	Set 5	Set 6
	Reps						
	Weight						
	Reps						
	Weight						
	Reps						
	Weight						
	Reps						
	Weight						
	Reps						
	Weight						
	Reps						
	Weight						
	Reps						
	Weight						
	Reps						
	Weight						
	Reps						
	Weight						
	Reps						
	Weight						

Cardio

Exercise	Calories	Distance	Time

Water Intake _____________________

Cooldown _____________________

Feeling ☆ ☆ ☆ ☆ ☆

Notes

Today's Goal　＿＿＿＿＿＿　Ⓜ Ⓣ Ⓦ Ⓣ Ⓕ Ⓢ Ⓢ

Muscle Group Focus ＿＿＿＿＿　Weight ＿＿＿＿　Date/Time ＿＿＿＿＿

Stretch ◯　Warm-Up ＿＿＿＿＿＿＿＿＿＿＿＿＿＿＿＿＿

Strength Training

Exercise		Set 1	Set 2	Set 3	Set 4	Set 5	Set 6
	Reps						
	Weight						
	Reps						
	Weight						
	Reps						
	Weight						
	Reps						
	Weight						
	Reps						
	Weight						
	Reps						
	Weight						
	Reps						
	Weight						
	Reps						
	Weight						
	Reps						
	Weight						

Cardio

Exercise	Calories	Distance	Time

Water Intake ＿＿＿＿＿＿＿＿＿＿＿

Cooldown ＿＿＿＿＿＿＿＿＿

Feeling ☆ ☆ ☆ ☆ ☆

Notes

Today's Goal _____________   Ⓜ Ⓣ Ⓦ Ⓣ Ⓕ Ⓢ Ⓢ

Muscle Group Focus _________   Weight ________   Date/Time __________

Stretch ◯   Warm-Up _______________________________

Strength Training

Exercise		Set 1	Set 2	Set 3	Set 4	Set 5	Set 6
	Reps						
	Weight						
	Reps						
	Weight						
	Reps						
	Weight						
	Reps						
	Weight						
	Reps						
	Weight						
	Reps						
	Weight						
	Reps						
	Weight						
	Reps						
	Weight						
	Reps						
	Weight						
	Reps						
	Weight						

Cardio

Exercise	Calories	Distance	Time

Water Intake _______________

Cooldown _______________

Feeling ☆ ☆ ☆ ☆ ☆

Notes

Today's Goal   (M) (T) (W) (T) (F) (S) (S)

Muscle Group Focus _________   Weight _______   Date/Time _________

Stretch ◯   Warm-Up ________________________________

Strength Training

Exercise		Set 1	Set 2	Set 3	Set 4	Set 5	Set 6
	Reps						
	Weight						
	Reps						
	Weight						
	Reps						
	Weight						
	Reps						
	Weight						
	Reps						
	Weight						
	Reps						
	Weight						
	Reps						
	Weight						
	Reps						
	Weight						
	Reps						
	Weight						
	Reps						
	Weight						

Cardio

Exercise	Calories	Distance	Time

Water Intake ________________

Cooldown ________________

Feeling ☆ ☆ ☆ ☆ ☆

Notes

Today's Goal _______________ (M) (T) (W) (T) (F) **(S)** **(S)**

Muscle Group Focus _________ Weight ________ Date/Time _________

Stretch ◯ Warm-Up _______________________________

Strength Training

Exercise		Set 1	Set 2	Set 3	Set 4	Set 5	Set 6
	Reps						
	Weight						
	Reps						
	Weight						
	Reps						
	Weight						
	Reps						
	Weight						
	Reps						
	Weight						
	Reps						
	Weight						
	Reps						
	Weight						
	Reps						
	Weight						
	Reps						
	Weight						
	Reps						
	Weight						

Cardio

Exercise	Calories	Distance	Time

Water Intake _______________

Cooldown _______________

Feeling ☆ ☆ ☆ ☆ ☆

Notes

Today's Goal   _____________   (M) (T) (W) (T) (F) **S** **S**

Muscle Group Focus __________   Weight ________   Date/Time __________

Stretch ◯   Warm-Up ________________________________

Strength Training

Exercise		Set 1	Set 2	Set 3	Set 4	Set 5	Set 6
	Reps						
	Weight						
	Reps						
	Weight						
	Reps						
	Weight						
	Reps						
	Weight						
	Reps						
	Weight						
	Reps						
	Weight						
	Reps						
	Weight						
	Reps						
	Weight						
	Reps						
	Weight						

Cardio

Exercise	Calories	Distance	Time

Water Intake ________________

Cooldown ________________

Feeling ☆ ☆ ☆ ☆ ☆

Notes

Today's Goal _______________ Ⓜ Ⓣ Ⓦ Ⓣ Ⓕ ⚫S ⚫S

Muscle Group Focus ___________   Weight ________   Date/Time ___________

Stretch ◯   Warm-Up _______________________________

Strength Training

Exercise		Set 1	Set 2	Set 3	Set 4	Set 5	Set 6
	Reps						
	Weight						
	Reps						
	Weight						
	Reps						
	Weight						
	Reps						
	Weight						
	Reps						
	Weight						
	Reps						
	Weight						
	Reps						
	Weight						
	Reps						
	Weight						
	Reps						
	Weight						
	Reps						
	Weight						

Cardio

Exercise	Calories	Distance	Time

Water Intake _______________

Cooldown _______________

Feeling ☆ ☆ ☆ ☆ ☆

Notes

Today's Goal ___________ (M) (T) (W) (T) (F) **(S)** **(S)**

Muscle Group Focus ___________   Weight _______   Date/Time ___________

Stretch ◯   Warm-Up ___________________________________

Strength Training

Exercise		Set 1	Set 2	Set 3	Set 4	Set 5	Set 6
	Reps						
	Weight						
	Reps						
	Weight						
	Reps						
	Weight						
	Reps						
	Weight						
	Reps						
	Weight						
	Reps						
	Weight						
	Reps						
	Weight						
	Reps						
	Weight						
	Reps						
	Weight						
	Reps						
	Weight						

Cardio

Exercise	Calories	Distance	Time

Water Intake ___________

Cooldown ___________

Feeling ☆ ☆ ☆ ☆ ☆

Notes

Today's Goal _____________   (M) (T) (W) (T) (F) (S) (S)

Muscle Group Focus __________   Weight _________   Date/Time ___________

Stretch ◯   Warm-Up ____

Strength Training

Exercise		Set 1	Set 2	Set 3	Set 4	Set 5	Set 6
	Reps						
	Weight						
	Reps						
	Weight						
	Reps						
	Weight						
	Reps						
	Weight						
	Reps						
	Weight						
	Reps						
	Weight						
	Reps						
	Weight						
	Reps						
	Weight						
	Reps						
	Weight						
	Reps						
	Weight						

Cardio

Exercise	Calories	Distance	Time

Water Intake _________________

Cooldown _________________

Feeling ☆ ☆ ☆ ☆ ☆

Notes

Today's Goal _____________ Ⓜ Ⓣ Ⓦ Ⓣ Ⓕ ⬤S ⬤S

Muscle Group Focus __________   Weight _______   Date/Time __________

Stretch ◯   Warm-Up ________________________________

Strength Training

Exercise		Set 1	Set 2	Set 3	Set 4	Set 5	Set 6
	Reps						
	Weight						
	Reps						
	Weight						
	Reps						
	Weight						
	Reps						
	Weight						
	Reps						
	Weight						
	Reps						
	Weight						
	Reps						
	Weight						
	Reps						
	Weight						
	Reps						
	Weight						

Cardio

Exercise	Calories	Distance	Time

Water Intake __________________

Cooldown __________________

Feeling ☆ ☆ ☆ ☆ ☆

Notes

Today's Goal ___________ (M) (T) (W) (T) (F) (S) (S)

Muscle Group Focus __________   Weight _________   Date/Time ___________

Stretch ◯   Warm-Up ___________________________________

Strength Training

Exercise		Set 1	Set 2	Set 3	Set 4	Set 5	Set 6
	Reps						
	Weight						
	Reps						
	Weight						
	Reps						
	Weight						
	Reps						
	Weight						
	Reps						
	Weight						
	Reps						
	Weight						
	Reps						
	Weight						
	Reps						
	Weight						
	Reps						
	Weight						

Cardio

Exercise	Calories	Distance	Time

Water Intake ___________________

Cooldown ___________

Feeling ☆ ☆ ☆ ☆ ☆

Notes

Today's Goal ____________   Ⓜ Ⓣ Ⓦ Ⓣ Ⓕ ⬤S ⬤S

Muscle Group Focus ___________   Weight ________   Date/Time __________

Stretch ◯   Warm-Up ____

Strength Training

Exercise		Set 1	Set 2	Set 3	Set 4	Set 5	Set 6
	Reps						
	Weight						
	Reps						
	Weight						
	Reps						
	Weight						
	Reps						
	Weight						
	Reps						
	Weight						
	Reps						
	Weight						
	Reps						
	Weight						
	Reps						
	Weight						
	Reps						
	Weight						
	Reps						
	Weight						

Cardio

Exercise	Calories	Distance	Time

Water Intake ________________

Cooldown ________________

Feeling ☆ ☆ ☆ ☆ ☆

Notes

Today's Goal __________   Ⓜ Ⓣ Ⓦ Ⓣ Ⓕ Ⓢ Ⓢ

Muscle Group Focus __________   Weight __________   Date/Time __________

Stretch ◯   Warm-Up __________

Strength Training

Exercise		Set 1	Set 2	Set 3	Set 4	Set 5	Set 6
	Reps						
	Weight						
	Reps						
	Weight						
	Reps						
	Weight						
	Reps						
	Weight						
	Reps						
	Weight						
	Reps						
	Weight						
	Reps						
	Weight						
	Reps						
	Weight						
	Reps						
	Weight						

Cardio

Exercise	Calories	Distance	Time

Water Intake __________

Cooldown __________

Feeling ☆ ☆ ☆ ☆ ☆

Notes

Today's Goal ____________   Ⓜ Ⓣ Ⓦ Ⓣ Ⓕ ⬤S ⬤S

Muscle Group Focus __________   Weight ________   Date/Time __________

Stretch ◯   Warm-Up ____________________________________

Strength Training

Exercise		Set 1	Set 2	Set 3	Set 4	Set 5	Set 6
	Reps						
	Weight						
	Reps						
	Weight						
	Reps						
	Weight						
	Reps						
	Weight						
	Reps						
	Weight						
	Reps						
	Weight						
	Reps						
	Weight						
	Reps						
	Weight						
	Reps						
	Weight						
	Reps						
	Weight						

Cardio

Exercise	Calories	Distance	Time

Water Intake ____________

Cooldown ____________

Feeling ☆ ☆ ☆ ☆ ☆

Notes

Today's Goal ___________   (M) (T) (W) (T) (F) (S) (S)

Muscle Group Focus ___________   Weight ________   Date/Time ___________

Stretch ◯   Warm-Up ___________________________________

Strength Training

Exercise		Set 1	Set 2	Set 3	Set 4	Set 5	Set 6
	Reps						
	Weight						
	Reps						
	Weight						
	Reps						
	Weight						
	Reps						
	Weight						
	Reps						
	Weight						
	Reps						
	Weight						
	Reps						
	Weight						
	Reps						
	Weight						
	Reps						
	Weight						
	Reps						
	Weight						

Cardio

Exercise	Calories	Distance	Time

Water Intake ___________________

Cooldown ___________________

Feeling ☆ ☆ ☆ ☆ ☆

Notes

Today's Goal ____________   Ⓜ Ⓣ Ⓦ Ⓣ Ⓕ ⬤S ⬤S

Muscle Group Focus _________ Weight _______ Date/Time __________

Stretch ◯   Warm-Up ___________________________________

Strength Training

Exercise		Set 1	Set 2	Set 3	Set 4	Set 5	Set 6
	Reps						
	Weight						
	Reps						
	Weight						
	Reps						
	Weight						
	Reps						
	Weight						
	Reps						
	Weight						
	Reps						
	Weight						
	Reps						
	Weight						
	Reps						
	Weight						
	Reps						
	Weight						
	Reps						
	Weight						

Cardio

Exercise	Calories	Distance	Time

Water Intake ___________________

Cooldown _________________

Feeling ☆ ☆ ☆ ☆ ☆

Notes

Today's Goal ____________   (M) (T) (W) (T) (F) (S) (S)

Muscle Group Focus ____________   Weight ________   Date/Time ____________

Stretch ◯   Warm-Up ____________

Strength Training

Exercise		Set 1	Set 2	Set 3	Set 4	Set 5	Set 6
	Reps						
	Weight						
	Reps						
	Weight						
	Reps						
	Weight						
	Reps						
	Weight						
	Reps						
	Weight						
	Reps						
	Weight						
	Reps						
	Weight						
	Reps						
	Weight						
	Reps						
	Weight						

Cardio

Exercise	Calories	Distance	Time

Water Intake ____________

Cooldown ____________

Feeling ☆ ☆ ☆ ☆ ☆

Notes

Today's Goal ___________   Ⓜ Ⓣ Ⓦ Ⓣ Ⓕ ⚫S ⚫S

Muscle Group Focus __________   Weight ________   Date/Time __________

Stretch ◯   Warm-Up _______________________________

Strength Training

Exercise		Set 1	Set 2	Set 3	Set 4	Set 5	Set 6
	Reps						
	Weight						
	Reps						
	Weight						
	Reps						
	Weight						
	Reps						
	Weight						
	Reps						
	Weight						
	Reps						
	Weight						
	Reps						
	Weight						
	Reps						
	Weight						
	Reps						
	Weight						
	Reps						
	Weight						

Cardio

Exercise	Calories	Distance	Time

Water Intake _______________

Cooldown _______________

Feeling ☆ ☆ ☆ ☆ ☆

Notes

Today's Goal _____ (M) (T) (W) (T) (F) (S) (S)

Muscle Group Focus _____ Weight _____ Date/Time _____

Stretch ◯   Warm-Up _____

Strength Training

Exercise		Set 1	Set 2	Set 3	Set 4	Set 5	Set 6
	Reps						
	Weight						
	Reps						
	Weight						
	Reps						
	Weight						
	Reps						
	Weight						
	Reps						
	Weight						
	Reps						
	Weight						
	Reps						
	Weight						
	Reps						
	Weight						
	Reps						
	Weight						

Cardio

Exercise	Calories	Distance	Time

Water Intake _____

Cooldown _____

Feeling ☆ ☆ ☆ ☆ ☆

Notes

Today's Goal ___________ Ⓜ Ⓣ Ⓦ Ⓣ Ⓕ ⚫S ⚫S

Muscle Group Focus ___________ Weight ________ Date/Time ___________

Stretch ◯   Warm-Up ___________________________________

Strength Training

Exercise		Set 1	Set 2	Set 3	Set 4	Set 5	Set 6
	Reps						
	Weight						
	Reps						
	Weight						
	Reps						
	Weight						
	Reps						
	Weight						
	Reps						
	Weight						
	Reps						
	Weight						
	Reps						
	Weight						
	Reps						
	Weight						

Cardio

Exercise	Calories	Distance	Time

Water Intake ___________

Cooldown ___________

Feeling ☆ ☆ ☆ ☆ ☆

Notes

Today's Goal ___________   Ⓜ Ⓣ Ⓦ Ⓣ Ⓕ Ⓢ Ⓢ

Muscle Group Focus __________   Weight ________   Date/Time __________

Stretch ◯   Warm-Up ________________________________

Strength Training

Exercise		Set 1	Set 2	Set 3	Set 4	Set 5	Set 6
	Reps						
	Weight						
	Reps						
	Weight						
	Reps						
	Weight						
	Reps						
	Weight						
	Reps						
	Weight						
	Reps						
	Weight						
	Reps						
	Weight						
	Reps						
	Weight						
	Reps						
	Weight						
	Reps						
	Weight						

Cardio

Exercise	Calories	Distance	Time

Water Intake ________________

Cooldown ________________

Feeling ☆ ☆ ☆ ☆ ☆

Notes

Today's Goal ______________   (M) (T) (W) (T) (F) (S) (S)

Muscle Group Focus __________   Weight ________   Date/Time __________

Stretch ◯   Warm-Up ________________________________

Strength Training

Exercise		Set 1	Set 2	Set 3	Set 4	Set 5	Set 6
	Reps						
	Weight						
	Reps						
	Weight						
	Reps						
	Weight						
	Reps						
	Weight						
	Reps						
	Weight						
	Reps						
	Weight						
	Reps						
	Weight						
	Reps						
	Weight						
	Reps						
	Weight						
	Reps						
	Weight						

Cardio

Exercise	Calories	Distance	Time

Water Intake __________

Cooldown __________

Feeling ☆ ☆ ☆ ☆ ☆

Notes

Today's Goal ___________ (M) (T) (W) (T) (F) (S) (S)

Muscle Group Focus ___________   Weight _______   Date/Time ___________

Stretch ◯   Warm-Up ___________________________________

Strength Training

Exercise		Set 1	Set 2	Set 3	Set 4	Set 5	Set 6
	Reps						
	Weight						
	Reps						
	Weight						
	Reps						
	Weight						
	Reps						
	Weight						
	Reps						
	Weight						
	Reps						
	Weight						
	Reps						
	Weight						
	Reps						
	Weight						
	Reps						
	Weight						

Cardio

Exercise	Calories	Distance	Time

Water Intake ___________

Cooldown ___________

Feeling ☆ ☆ ☆ ☆ ☆

Notes

Today's Goal _______   Ⓜ Ⓣ Ⓦ Ⓣ Ⓕ Ⓢ Ⓢ

Muscle Group Focus _______   Weight _______   Date/Time _______

Stretch ◯   Warm-Up _______________________________

Strength Training

Exercise		Set 1	Set 2	Set 3	Set 4	Set 5	Set 6
	Reps						
	Weight						
	Reps						
	Weight						
	Reps						
	Weight						
	Reps						
	Weight						
	Reps						
	Weight						
	Reps						
	Weight						
	Reps						
	Weight						
	Reps						
	Weight						
	Reps						
	Weight						
	Reps						
	Weight						

Cardio

Exercise	Calories	Distance	Time

Water Intake _______________

Cooldown _______________

Feeling ☆ ☆ ☆ ☆ ☆

Notes

Today's Goal _____________   Ⓜ Ⓣ Ⓦ Ⓣ Ⓕ ⬤S ⬤S

Muscle Group Focus __________   Weight _________   Date/Time ___________

Stretch ◯   Warm-Up ____

Strength Training

Exercise		Set 1	Set 2	Set 3	Set 4	Set 5	Set 6
	Reps						
	Weight						
	Reps						
	Weight						
	Reps						
	Weight						
	Reps						
	Weight						
	Reps						
	Weight						
	Reps						
	Weight						
	Reps						
	Weight						
	Reps						
	Weight						
	Reps						
	Weight						
	Reps						
	Weight						

Cardio

Exercise	Calories	Distance	Time

Water Intake _________________

Cooldown _________________

Feeling ☆ ☆ ☆ ☆ ☆

Notes

Today's Goal _______ Ⓜ Ⓣ Ⓦ Ⓣ Ⓕ ● ●

Muscle Group Focus _______   Weight _______   Date/Time _______

Stretch ◯   Warm-Up _______________________________

Strength Training

Exercise		Set 1	Set 2	Set 3	Set 4	Set 5	Set 6
	Reps						
	Weight						
	Reps						
	Weight						
	Reps						
	Weight						
	Reps						
	Weight						
	Reps						
	Weight						
	Reps						
	Weight						
	Reps						
	Weight						
	Reps						
	Weight						

Cardio

Exercise	Calories	Distance	Time

Water Intake _______________

Cooldown _______________

Feeling ☆ ☆ ☆ ☆ ☆

Notes

Today's Goal __________   (M) (T) (W) (T) (F) (S) (S)

Muscle Group Focus __________   Weight ________   Date/Time __________

Stretch ◯   Warm-Up __________________________

Strength Training

Exercise		Set 1	Set 2	Set 3	Set 4	Set 5	Set 6
	Reps						
	Weight						
	Reps						
	Weight						
	Reps						
	Weight						
	Reps						
	Weight						
	Reps						
	Weight						
	Reps						
	Weight						
	Reps						
	Weight						
	Reps						
	Weight						
	Reps						
	Weight						
	Reps						
	Weight						

Cardio

Exercise	Calories	Distance	Time

Water Intake __________________

Cooldown __________________

Feeling ☆ ☆ ☆ ☆ ☆

Notes

Today's Goal ___________   (M) (T) (W) (T) (F) (S) (S)

Muscle Group Focus ___________   Weight ________   Date/Time ___________

Stretch ◯   Warm-Up ____________________________________

Strength Training

Exercise		Set 1	Set 2	Set 3	Set 4	Set 5	Set 6
	Reps						
	Weight						
	Reps						
	Weight						
	Reps						
	Weight						
	Reps						
	Weight						
	Reps						
	Weight						
	Reps						
	Weight						
	Reps						
	Weight						
	Reps						
	Weight						
	Reps						
	Weight						
	Reps						
	Weight						

Cardio

Exercise	Calories	Distance	Time

Water Intake ____________________

Cooldown ____________________

Feeling ☆ ☆ ☆ ☆ ☆

Notes

Today's Goal ______   M T W T F **S** **S**

Muscle Group Focus ______   Weight ______   Date/Time ______

Stretch ◯   Warm-Up ______________

Strength Training

Exercise		Set 1	Set 2	Set 3	Set 4	Set 5	Set 6
	Reps						
	Weight						
	Reps						
	Weight						
	Reps						
	Weight						
	Reps						
	Weight						
	Reps						
	Weight						
	Reps						
	Weight						
	Reps						
	Weight						
	Reps						
	Weight						
	Reps						
	Weight						
	Reps						
	Weight						

Cardio

Exercise	Calories	Distance	Time

Water Intake ______

Cooldown ______

Feeling ☆ ☆ ☆ ☆ ☆

Notes

Today's Goal _____________   Ⓜ Ⓣ Ⓦ Ⓣ Ⓕ Ⓢ Ⓢ

Muscle Group Focus __________   Weight ________   Date/Time __________

Stretch ◯   Warm-Up ________________________________

Strength Training

Exercise		Set 1	Set 2	Set 3	Set 4	Set 5	Set 6
	Reps						
	Weight						
	Reps						
	Weight						
	Reps						
	Weight						
	Reps						
	Weight						
	Reps						
	Weight						
	Reps						
	Weight						
	Reps						
	Weight						
	Reps						
	Weight						
	Reps						
	Weight						

Cardio

Exercise	Calories	Distance	Time

Water Intake ________________

Cooldown ________________

Feeling ☆ ☆ ☆ ☆ ☆

Notes

Today's Goal _____________   (M) (T) (W) (T) (F) (S) (S)

Muscle Group Focus _________   Weight ________   Date/Time __________

Stretch ◯   Warm-Up _________________________________

Strength Training

Exercise		Set 1	Set 2	Set 3	Set 4	Set 5	Set 6
	Reps						
	Weight						
	Reps						
	Weight						
	Reps						
	Weight						
	Reps						
	Weight						
	Reps						
	Weight						
	Reps						
	Weight						
	Reps						
	Weight						
	Reps						
	Weight						
	Reps						
	Weight						
	Reps						
	Weight						

Cardio

Exercise	Calories	Distance	Time

Water Intake _________________________

Cooldown _________________________

Feeling ☆ ☆ ☆ ☆ ☆

Notes

Today's Goal ____________   (M) (T) (W) (T) (F) (S) (S)

Muscle Group Focus __________   Weight _______   Date/Time __________

Stretch ◯   Warm-Up _____________________________________

Strength Training

Exercise		Set 1	Set 2	Set 3	Set 4	Set 5	Set 6
	Reps						
	Weight						
	Reps						
	Weight						
	Reps						
	Weight						
	Reps						
	Weight						
	Reps						
	Weight						
	Reps						
	Weight						
	Reps						
	Weight						
	Reps						
	Weight						
	Reps						
	Weight						
	Reps						
	Weight						

Cardio

Exercise	Calories	Distance	Time

Water Intake _________________________

Cooldown _________________________

Feeling ☆ ☆ ☆ ☆ ☆

Notes

Today's Goal ___________ (M) (T) (W) (T) (F) (S) (S)

Muscle Group Focus ___________   Weight _________   Date/Time ___________

Stretch ◯   Warm-Up ___________________________________

Strength Training

Exercise		Set 1	Set 2	Set 3	Set 4	Set 5	Set 6
	Reps						
	Weight						
	Reps						
	Weight						
	Reps						
	Weight						
	Reps						
	Weight						
	Reps						
	Weight						
	Reps						
	Weight						
	Reps						
	Weight						
	Reps						
	Weight						
	Reps						
	Weight						
	Reps						
	Weight						

Cardio

Exercise	Calories	Distance	Time

Water Intake ___________

Cooldown ___________

Feeling ☆ ☆ ☆ ☆ ☆

Notes

Today's Goal ____________ (M) (T) (W) (T) (F) (S) (S)

Muscle Group Focus __________   Weight ________   Date/Time __________

Stretch ○   Warm-Up ____

Strength Training

Exercise		Set 1	Set 2	Set 3	Set 4	Set 5	Set 6
	Reps						
	Weight						
	Reps						
	Weight						
	Reps						
	Weight						
	Reps						
	Weight						
	Reps						
	Weight						
	Reps						
	Weight						
	Reps						
	Weight						
	Reps						
	Weight						
	Reps						
	Weight						

Cardio

Exercise	Calories	Distance	Time

Water Intake ________________

Cooldown ________________

Feeling ☆ ☆ ☆ ☆ ☆

Notes

Today's Goal ______________ Ⓜ Ⓣ Ⓦ Ⓣ Ⓕ Ⓢ Ⓢ

Muscle Group Focus ___________ Weight ________ Date/Time __________

Stretch ◯   Warm-Up ____

Strength Training

Exercise		Set 1	Set 2	Set 3	Set 4	Set 5	Set 6
	Reps						
	Weight						
	Reps						
	Weight						
	Reps						
	Weight						
	Reps						
	Weight						
	Reps						
	Weight						
	Reps						
	Weight						
	Reps						
	Weight						
	Reps						
	Weight						
	Reps						
	Weight						
	Reps						
	Weight						

Cardio

Exercise	Calories	Distance	Time

Water Intake ____________________

Cooldown ____________________

Feeling ☆ ☆ ☆ ☆ ☆

Notes

Today's Goal ____________ Ⓜ Ⓣ Ⓦ Ⓣ Ⓕ ⬤S ⬤S

Muscle Group Focus __________ Weight ________ Date/Time __________

Stretch ◯ Warm-Up ________________________________

Strength Training

Exercise		Set 1	Set 2	Set 3	Set 4	Set 5	Set 6
	Reps						
	Weight						
	Reps						
	Weight						
	Reps						
	Weight						
	Reps						
	Weight						
	Reps						
	Weight						
	Reps						
	Weight						
	Reps						
	Weight						
	Reps						
	Weight						
	Reps						
	Weight						
	Reps						
	Weight						

Cardio

Exercise	Calories	Distance	Time

Water Intake ____________

Cooldown ____________

Feeling ☆ ☆ ☆ ☆ ☆

Notes

Today's Goal ______________   Ⓜ Ⓣ Ⓦ Ⓣ Ⓕ ⬤S ⬤S

Muscle Group Focus ___________   Weight ________   Date/Time ___________

Stretch ◯   Warm-Up ___________________________________

Strength Training

Exercise		Set 1	Set 2	Set 3	Set 4	Set 5	Set 6
	Reps						
	Weight						
	Reps						
	Weight						
	Reps						
	Weight						
	Reps						
	Weight						
	Reps						
	Weight						
	Reps						
	Weight						
	Reps						
	Weight						
	Reps						
	Weight						
	Reps						
	Weight						
	Reps						
	Weight						

Cardio

Exercise	Calories	Distance	Time

Water Intake ___________________

Cooldown ___________________

Feeling ☆ ☆ ☆ ☆ ☆

Notes

Today's Goal ____________   M T W T F S S

Muscle Group Focus __________   Weight ________   Date/Time __________

Stretch ◯   Warm-Up ____

Strength Training

Exercise		Set 1	Set 2	Set 3	Set 4	Set 5	Set 6
	Reps						
	Weight						
	Reps						
	Weight						
	Reps						
	Weight						
	Reps						
	Weight						
	Reps						
	Weight						
	Reps						
	Weight						
	Reps						
	Weight						
	Reps						
	Weight						
	Reps						
	Weight						
	Reps						
	Weight						

Cardio

Exercise	Calories	Distance	Time

Water Intake ________________

Cooldown ________________

Feeling ☆ ☆ ☆ ☆ ☆

Notes

Today's Goal ________   Ⓜ Ⓣ Ⓦ Ⓣ Ⓕ ⬤S ⬤S

Muscle Group Focus _________   Weight ________   Date/Time _________

Stretch ◯   Warm-Up ____________________________

Strength Training

Exercise		Set 1	Set 2	Set 3	Set 4	Set 5	Set 6
	Reps						
	Weight						
	Reps						
	Weight						
	Reps						
	Weight						
	Reps						
	Weight						
	Reps						
	Weight						
	Reps						
	Weight						
	Reps						
	Weight						
	Reps						
	Weight						
	Reps						
	Weight						
	Reps						
	Weight						

Cardio

Exercise	Calories	Distance	Time

Water Intake ________________

Cooldown ________________

Feeling ☆ ☆ ☆ ☆ ☆

Notes

Today's Goal ______________   Ⓜ Ⓣ Ⓦ Ⓣ Ⓕ ⬤S ⬤S

Muscle Group Focus __________   Weight ________   Date/Time ____________

Stretch ◯   Warm-Up ________________________________

Strength Training

Exercise		Set 1	Set 2	Set 3	Set 4	Set 5	Set 6
	Reps						
	Weight						
	Reps						
	Weight						
	Reps						
	Weight						
	Reps						
	Weight						
	Reps						
	Weight						
	Reps						
	Weight						
	Reps						
	Weight						
	Reps						
	Weight						
	Reps						
	Weight						
	Reps						
	Weight						

Cardio

Exercise	Calories	Distance	Time

Water Intake ________________

Cooldown ________________

Feeling ☆ ☆ ☆ ☆ ☆

Notes

Today's Goal ________   Ⓜ Ⓣ Ⓦ Ⓣ Ⓕ Ⓢ Ⓢ

Muscle Group Focus ________   Weight ________   Date/Time ________

Stretch ◯   Warm-Up ________________________

Strength Training

Exercise		Set 1	Set 2	Set 3	Set 4	Set 5	Set 6
	Reps						
	Weight						
	Reps						
	Weight						
	Reps						
	Weight						
	Reps						
	Weight						
	Reps						
	Weight						
	Reps						
	Weight						
	Reps						
	Weight						
	Reps						
	Weight						
	Reps						
	Weight						
	Reps						
	Weight						

Cardio

Exercise	Calories	Distance	Time

Water Intake ________________

Cooldown ________________

Feeling ☆ ☆ ☆ ☆ ☆

Notes

Today's Goal _____________   Ⓜ Ⓣ Ⓦ Ⓣ Ⓕ ⬤S ⬤S

Muscle Group Focus ___________   Weight ________   Date/Time __________

Stretch ◯   Warm-Up ___________________________________

Strength Training

Exercise		Set 1	Set 2	Set 3	Set 4	Set 5	Set 6
	Reps						
	Weight						
	Reps						
	Weight						
	Reps						
	Weight						
	Reps						
	Weight						
	Reps						
	Weight						
	Reps						
	Weight						
	Reps						
	Weight						
	Reps						
	Weight						
	Reps						
	Weight						
	Reps						
	Weight						

Cardio

Exercise	Calories	Distance	Time

Water Intake ___________________

Cooldown ___________________

Feeling ☆ ☆ ☆ ☆ ☆

Notes

Today's Goal ____________   Ⓜ Ⓣ Ⓦ Ⓣ Ⓕ ⬤S ⬤S

Muscle Group Focus __________   Weight ________   Date/Time ____________

Stretch ◯   Warm-Up ____

Strength Training

Exercise		Set 1	Set 2	Set 3	Set 4	Set 5	Set 6
	Reps						
	Weight						
	Reps						
	Weight						
	Reps						
	Weight						
	Reps						
	Weight						
	Reps						
	Weight						
	Reps						
	Weight						
	Reps						
	Weight						
	Reps						
	Weight						
	Reps						
	Weight						
	Reps						
	Weight						

Cardio

Exercise	Calories	Distance	Time

Water Intake ____________________

Cooldown ____________________

Feeling ☆ ☆ ☆ ☆ ☆

Notes

Today's Goal _____________   (M) (T) (W) (T) (F) (S) (S)

Muscle Group Focus __________   Weight ________   Date/Time __________

Stretch ◯   Warm-Up _____________________________________

Strength Training

Exercise		Set 1	Set 2	Set 3	Set 4	Set 5	Set 6
	Reps						
	Weight						
	Reps						
	Weight						
	Reps						
	Weight						
	Reps						
	Weight						
	Reps						
	Weight						
	Reps						
	Weight						
	Reps						
	Weight						
	Reps						
	Weight						
	Reps						
	Weight						

Cardio

Exercise	Calories	Distance	Time

Water Intake _____________

Cooldown _____________

Feeling ☆ ☆ ☆ ☆ ☆

Notes

Today's Goal ____________ (M) (T) (W) (T) (F) (S) (S)

Muscle Group Focus __________ Weight ________ Date/Time __________

Stretch ◯   Warm-Up ____

Strength Training

Exercise		Set 1	Set 2	Set 3	Set 4	Set 5	Set 6
	Reps						
	Weight						
	Reps						
	Weight						
	Reps						
	Weight						
	Reps						
	Weight						
	Reps						
	Weight						
	Reps						
	Weight						
	Reps						
	Weight						
	Reps						
	Weight						
	Reps						
	Weight						

Cardio

Exercise	Calories	Distance	Time

Water Intake ________________

Cooldown ________________

Feeling ☆ ☆ ☆ ☆ ☆

Notes

Today's Goal _____________   (M) (T) (W) (T) (F) (S) (S)

Muscle Group Focus __________   Weight ________   Date/Time ___________

Stretch ◯   Warm-Up ________________________________

Strength Training

Exercise		Set 1	Set 2	Set 3	Set 4	Set 5	Set 6
	Reps						
	Weight						
	Reps						
	Weight						
	Reps						
	Weight						
	Reps						
	Weight						
	Reps						
	Weight						
	Reps						
	Weight						
	Reps						
	Weight						
	Reps						
	Weight						
	Reps						
	Weight						
	Reps						
	Weight						

Cardio

Exercise	Calories	Distance	Time

Water Intake ________________

Cooldown ________________

Feeling ☆ ☆ ☆ ☆ ☆

Notes

Today's Goal ____________ (M) (T) (W) (T) (F) (S) (S)

Muscle Group Focus __________   Weight ________   Date/Time __________

Stretch ◯   Warm-Up ________________________________

Strength Training

Exercise		Set 1	Set 2	Set 3	Set 4	Set 5	Set 6
	Reps						
	Weight						
	Reps						
	Weight						
	Reps						
	Weight						
	Reps						
	Weight						
	Reps						
	Weight						
	Reps						
	Weight						
	Reps						
	Weight						
	Reps						
	Weight						
	Reps						
	Weight						
	Reps						
	Weight						

Cardio

Exercise	Calories	Distance	Time

Water Intake ________________

Cooldown ________________

Feeling ☆ ☆ ☆ ☆ ☆

Notes

Today's Goal   __________   (M) (T) (W) (T) (F) (S) (S)

Muscle Group Focus __________   Weight _______   Date/Time __________

Stretch ◯   Warm-Up __________________________________

Strength Training

Exercise		Set 1	Set 2	Set 3	Set 4	Set 5	Set 6
	Reps						
	Weight						
	Reps						
	Weight						
	Reps						
	Weight						
	Reps						
	Weight						
	Reps						
	Weight						
	Reps						
	Weight						
	Reps						
	Weight						
	Reps						
	Weight						
	Reps						
	Weight						
	Reps						
	Weight						

Cardio

Exercise	Calories	Distance	Time

Water Intake __________________

Cooldown __________________

Feeling ☆ ☆ ☆ ☆ ☆

Notes

Today's Goal _____________ Ⓜ Ⓣ Ⓦ Ⓣ Ⓕ ⬤S ⬤S

Muscle Group Focus ___________   Weight ________   Date/Time ___________

Stretch ◯   Warm-Up ____

Strength Training

Exercise		Set 1	Set 2	Set 3	Set 4	Set 5	Set 6
	Reps						
	Weight						
	Reps						
	Weight						
	Reps						
	Weight						
	Reps						
	Weight						
	Reps						
	Weight						
	Reps						
	Weight						
	Reps						
	Weight						
	Reps						
	Weight						
	Reps						
	Weight						
	Reps						
	Weight						

Cardio

Exercise	Calories	Distance	Time

Water Intake _________________

Cooldown _________________

Feeling ☆ ☆ ☆ ☆ ☆

Notes

Today's Goal _____________ Ⓜ Ⓣ Ⓦ Ⓣ Ⓕ ⬤S ⬤S

Muscle Group Focus __________   Weight ________   Date/Time __________

Stretch ◯   Warm-Up ________________________________

Strength Training

Exercise		Set 1	Set 2	Set 3	Set 4	Set 5	Set 6
	Reps						
	Weight						
	Reps						
	Weight						
	Reps						
	Weight						
	Reps						
	Weight						
	Reps						
	Weight						
	Reps						
	Weight						
	Reps						
	Weight						
	Reps						
	Weight						
	Reps						
	Weight						
	Reps						
	Weight						

Cardio

Exercise	Calories	Distance	Time

Water Intake ________________

Cooldown ________________

Feeling ☆ ☆ ☆ ☆ ☆

Notes

Today's Goal ______________   (M) (T) (W) (T) (F) (S) (S)

Muscle Group Focus __________   Weight ________   Date/Time __________

Stretch ◯   Warm-Up ________________________________

Strength Training

Exercise		Set 1	Set 2	Set 3	Set 4	Set 5	Set 6
	Reps						
	Weight						
	Reps						
	Weight						
	Reps						
	Weight						
	Reps						
	Weight						
	Reps						
	Weight						
	Reps						
	Weight						
	Reps						
	Weight						
	Reps						
	Weight						
	Reps						
	Weight						
	Reps						
	Weight						

Cardio

Exercise	Calories	Distance	Time

Water Intake ________________

Cooldown ________________

Feeling ☆ ☆ ☆ ☆ ☆

Notes

Today's Goal ___________ Ⓜ Ⓣ Ⓦ Ⓣ Ⓕ ⚫S ⚫S

Muscle Group Focus ___________ Weight _______ Date/Time ___________

Stretch ◯   Warm-Up ____________________________

Strength Training

Exercise		Set 1	Set 2	Set 3	Set 4	Set 5	Set 6
	Reps						
	Weight						
	Reps						
	Weight						
	Reps						
	Weight						
	Reps						
	Weight						
	Reps						
	Weight						
	Reps						
	Weight						
	Reps						
	Weight						
	Reps						
	Weight						
	Reps						
	Weight						
	Reps						
	Weight						

Cardio

Exercise	Calories	Distance	Time

Water Intake ____________________

Cooldown ____________________

Feeling ☆ ☆ ☆ ☆ ☆

Notes

Today's Goal ___________ (M) (T) (W) (T) (F) **(S)** **(S)**

Muscle Group Focus __________ Weight ________ Date/Time __________

Stretch ◯   Warm-Up __________________________________

Strength Training

Exercise		Set 1	Set 2	Set 3	Set 4	Set 5	Set 6
	Reps						
	Weight						
	Reps						
	Weight						
	Reps						
	Weight						
	Reps						
	Weight						
	Reps						
	Weight						
	Reps						
	Weight						
	Reps						
	Weight						
	Reps						
	Weight						
	Reps						
	Weight						
	Reps						
	Weight						

Cardio

Exercise	Calories	Distance	Time

Water Intake __________

Cooldown __________

Feeling ☆ ☆ ☆ ☆ ☆

Notes

Today's Goal _____________   Ⓜ Ⓣ Ⓦ Ⓣ Ⓕ ⬤ ⬤

Muscle Group Focus __________   Weight ________   Date/Time __________

Stretch ◯   Warm-Up _______________________________________

Strength Training

Exercise		Set 1	Set 2	Set 3	Set 4	Set 5	Set 6
	Reps						
	Weight						
	Reps						
	Weight						
	Reps						
	Weight						
	Reps						
	Weight						
	Reps						
	Weight						
	Reps						
	Weight						
	Reps						
	Weight						
	Reps						
	Weight						
	Reps						
	Weight						
	Reps						
	Weight						

Cardio

Exercise	Calories	Distance	Time

Water Intake _______________

Cooldown _______________

Feeling ☆ ☆ ☆ ☆ ☆

Notes

Today's Goal ________________ Ⓜ Ⓣ Ⓦ Ⓣ Ⓕ Ⓢ Ⓢ

Muscle Group Focus __________   Weight ________   Date/Time __________

Stretch ◯   Warm-Up ________________________________

Strength Training

Exercise		Set 1	Set 2	Set 3	Set 4	Set 5	Set 6
	Reps						
	Weight						
	Reps						
	Weight						
	Reps						
	Weight						
	Reps						
	Weight						
	Reps						
	Weight						
	Reps						
	Weight						
	Reps						
	Weight						
	Reps						
	Weight						
	Reps						
	Weight						
	Reps						
	Weight						

Cardio

Exercise	Calories	Distance	Time

Water Intake ________________

Cooldown ________________

Feeling ☆ ☆ ☆ ☆ ☆

Notes

Today's Goal ________________ Ⓜ Ⓣ Ⓦ Ⓣ Ⓕ ⬤S ⬤S

Muscle Group Focus __________   Weight ________   Date/Time __________

Stretch ◯   Warm-Up ________________________________

Strength Training

Exercise		Set 1	Set 2	Set 3	Set 4	Set 5	Set 6
	Reps						
	Weight						
	Reps						
	Weight						
	Reps						
	Weight						
	Reps						
	Weight						
	Reps						
	Weight						
	Reps						
	Weight						
	Reps						
	Weight						
	Reps						
	Weight						
	Reps						
	Weight						
	Reps						
	Weight						

Cardio

Exercise	Calories	Distance	Time

Water Intake ________________

Cooldown ________________

Feeling ☆ ☆ ☆ ☆ ☆

Notes

Today's Goal ____________ (M) (T) (W) (T) (F) (S) (S)

Muscle Group Focus ________   Weight ________   Date/Time ________

Stretch ◯   Warm-Up ____________________________

Strength Training

Exercise		Set 1	Set 2	Set 3	Set 4	Set 5	Set 6
	Reps						
	Weight						
	Reps						
	Weight						
	Reps						
	Weight						
	Reps						
	Weight						
	Reps						
	Weight						
	Reps						
	Weight						
	Reps						
	Weight						
	Reps						
	Weight						
	Reps						
	Weight						
	Reps						
	Weight						

Cardio

Exercise	Calories	Distance	Time

Water Intake ____________

Cooldown ____________

Feeling ☆ ☆ ☆ ☆ ☆

Notes

Today's Goal _______________   (M) (T) (W) (T) (F) (S) (S)

Muscle Group Focus __________   Weight _______   Date/Time __________

Stretch ◯   Warm-Up _________________________________

Strength Training

Exercise		Set 1	Set 2	Set 3	Set 4	Set 5	Set 6
	Reps						
	Weight						
	Reps						
	Weight						
	Reps						
	Weight						
	Reps						
	Weight						
	Reps						
	Weight						
	Reps						
	Weight						
	Reps						
	Weight						
	Reps						
	Weight						
	Reps						
	Weight						
	Reps						
	Weight						

Cardio

Exercise	Calories	Distance	Time

Water Intake _________________

Cooldown _________________

Feeling ☆ ☆ ☆ ☆ ☆

Notes

Today's Goal ___________   Ⓜ Ⓣ Ⓦ Ⓣ Ⓕ ⚫ ⚫

Muscle Group Focus __________   Weight ________   Date/Time __________

Stretch ◯   Warm-Up ___________________________

Strength Training

Exercise		Set 1	Set 2	Set 3	Set 4	Set 5	Set 6
	Reps						
	Weight						
	Reps						
	Weight						
	Reps						
	Weight						
	Reps						
	Weight						
	Reps						
	Weight						
	Reps						
	Weight						
	Reps						
	Weight						
	Reps						
	Weight						
	Reps						
	Weight						
	Reps						
	Weight						

Cardio

Exercise	Calories	Distance	Time

Water Intake ___________________

Cooldown ___________________

Feeling ☆ ☆ ☆ ☆ ☆

Notes

Today's Goal _______________ Ⓜ Ⓣ Ⓦ Ⓣ Ⓕ ⬤S ⬤S

Muscle Group Focus __________ Weight ________ Date/Time __________

Stretch ◯   Warm-Up _______________________________

Strength Training

Exercise		Set 1	Set 2	Set 3	Set 4	Set 5	Set 6
	Reps						
	Weight						
	Reps						
	Weight						
	Reps						
	Weight						
	Reps						
	Weight						
	Reps						
	Weight						
	Reps						
	Weight						
	Reps						
	Weight						
	Reps						
	Weight						
	Reps						
	Weight						

Cardio

Exercise	Calories	Distance	Time

Water Intake _______________

Cooldown _______________

Feeling ☆ ☆ ☆ ☆ ☆

Notes

Today's Goal ___________ Ⓜ Ⓣ Ⓦ Ⓣ Ⓕ ⬤S ⬤S

Muscle Group Focus __________   Weight ________   Date/Time __________

Stretch ◯   Warm-Up ______________________________

Strength Training

Exercise		Set 1	Set 2	Set 3	Set 4	Set 5	Set 6
	Reps						
	Weight						
	Reps						
	Weight						
	Reps						
	Weight						
	Reps						
	Weight						
	Reps						
	Weight						
	Reps						
	Weight						
	Reps						
	Weight						
	Reps						
	Weight						
	Reps						
	Weight						
	Reps						
	Weight						

Cardio

Exercise	Calories	Distance	Time

Water Intake ______________

Cooldown ______________

Feeling ☆ ☆ ☆ ☆ ☆

Notes

Today's Goal ___________ (M) (T) (W) (T) (F) **(S) (S)**

Muscle Group Focus __________   Weight _______   Date/Time __________

Stretch ◯   Warm-Up ________________________

Strength Training

Exercise		Set 1	Set 2	Set 3	Set 4	Set 5	Set 6
	Reps						
	Weight						
	Reps						
	Weight						
	Reps						
	Weight						
	Reps						
	Weight						
	Reps						
	Weight						
	Reps						
	Weight						
	Reps						
	Weight						
	Reps						
	Weight						
	Reps						
	Weight						

Cardio

Exercise	Calories	Distance	Time

Water Intake ________________

Cooldown ________________

Feeling ☆ ☆ ☆ ☆ ☆

Notes